Introducing Self-Care

Self-care is essential for maintaining our overall well-being, encompassing various aspects of our lives. The practice involves intentionally prioritizing and attending to our physical, mental, emotional, social, and spiritual needs. In today's fast-paced world, where stress and responsibilities can easily take a toll on our health, practicing self-care and recognizing its importance is crucial.

Embark on a transformative journey of self-discovery and well-being with this meticulously-crafted self-care journal. Dive into enriching mental, emotional, social, spiritual, and physical self-care activities – each offering a unique pathway to inner harmony. Whether you choose to explore a daily practice from each category, or focus on one that resonates with you, this journal is your sacred space for personal growth.

Embrace the power of reflection, gratitude, and intentional living as you cultivate a balanced and resilient life. Remember, self-care is not a luxury, but a necessity for maintaining both mental and physical well-being. The journey begins with your pen and this journal – unlock the potential for a more mindful and fulfilling life today. Start journaling, and let the pages unfold your extraordinary story of self-care and joy!

Setting Goals

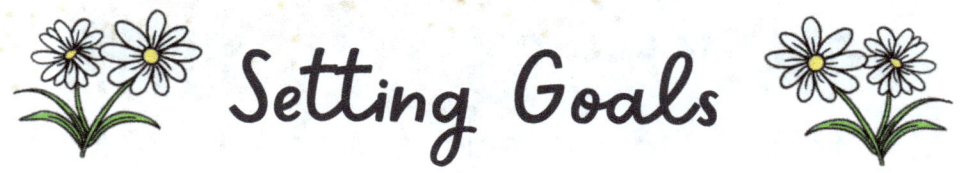

Setting goals across various areas of life is a transformative and empowering step. Articulating your aspirations helps pave the way for self-discovery and holistic growth. Writing down your goals acts as a compass, guiding you toward a more fulfilling and well-rounded life. Therefore, before you begin any self-care practices, take a few minutes to write down your goals. You can start by asking yourself questions such as, 'What do you want to improve in your life through self-care habits? How much time are you willing to spend daily on self-care practices?' Let's begin by writing down your goals for each category in the space provided.

Mental

....

....

....

....

....

Emotional

....
....
....
....
....

Social

....
....
....
....
....

Spiritual

....
....
....
....
....

Physical

....
....
....
....
....

 # Create A Routine

In this planner, you will be introduced to many different types of self-care practices. Take the time to experiment with each practice to find out which one is best for you. Feel free to modify or combine two or more practices to create a routine that suits you best. A daily self-care checklist is provided as a guide to keep track of your self-care practices.

Morning

- [ ] Wake up at _ _ _ am
- [ ] Drink a glass of water
- [ ] Make bed
- [ ] Breathe mindfully / meditate for 5 minutes
- [ ] Eat healthy breakfast

Throughout the Day

- [ ] Stay hydrated. Drink water regularly
- [ ] Eat nutritious meal
- [ ] Stretch / exercise
- [ ] Take warm bath / shower
- [ ] Engage in hobbies / creative activities

Before Sleep

- [ ] Limit screen time
- [ ] Wind down & declutter mind
- [ ] Sleep at _ _ _ pm

Work / School hours

- [ ] Prioritize tasks
- [ ] Create to-do lists
- [ ] Take short breaks
- [ ] Enjoy a calming tea / beverage

Find time to

- [ ] Call / communicate with friends / family
- [ ] Practice affirmations

Reflections

- [ ] Journal your thoughts / feelings
- [ ] Reflect on 5 things you're thankful for today
- [ ] Write down 3 things you achieved today
- [ ] Set intentions for the next day

Mental Self-Care

We can maintain a healthy mind by practicing mental self-care, which includes using mindfulness, stress management, and mental stimulation. Prioritizing our mental self-care will help safeguard our mental health, reduce anxiety, and enhance our quality of life.

Notes

....

....

....

....

....

....

....

....

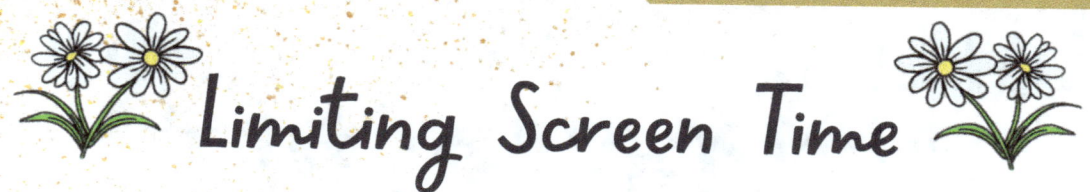

Limiting Screen Time

Excessive screen time can result in heightened stress levels, increased anxiety, and sleep disturbances. Limiting screen time can foster a calmer mental state, boost productivity, and promote mindful living. Utilize the provided table to log your screen time, facilitating an analysis of how much unnecessary time you spend on screens. This empowers you to plan and manage your screen time efficiently, fostering a more balanced and mindful daily routine.

Date	Device / platform	Start time	End time	Total time

Date	Device / platform	Start time	End time	Total time

Are there days when you are free from screen time? How does that make you feel?

....

....

....

....

....

....

....

Reading Daily

Engaging in daily reading is a powerful form of mental self-care. Reading allows the mind to temporarily detach from the pressures of daily life. It is good practice to read a few pages or engage in light reading each day. The provided table will assist you in planning your reading sessions.

📘 Book   🎧 Audiobook   📱 Digital

Title: ....

Author: ....   Genre: ....

Date started: ....   Progression: ....

Rating: ♡ ♡ ♡ ♡ ♡

What do you think of this book?

....

....

....

....

....

....

....

....

....

What is the most captivating aspect?

....

....

....

....

....

....

....

....

....

What did you learn from this book?

....

....

....

....

....

....

....

....

Book / Genre I want to read next: ....

 # Reading Daily

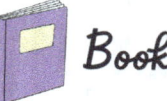 Book 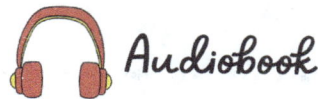 Audiobook Digital

Title: ....

Author: .... Genre: ....

Date started: .... Progression: ....

Rating: ♡ ♡ ♡ ♡ ♡

What do you think of this book?

....

....

....

....

....

....

....

....

....

....

What is the most captivating aspect?

....
....
....
....
....
....
....
....
....

What did you learn from this book?

....
....
....
....
....
....
....
....
....

Book / genre I want to read next: ....

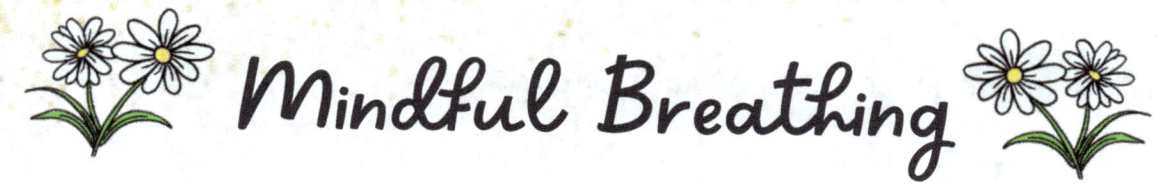

Mindful Breathing

Mindful breathing is a practice that directs focused attention to the breath, creating a sense of awareness in the present moment. This technique aids in detaching from the overwhelming stress and anxieties of daily challenges, enhancing mental wellness, and promoting a more peaceful state of mind. Try practicing mindful breathing for at least five minutes every day and record your thoughts before and after each session.

Date: ....

Duration: ....

How do you feel before your practice?

....

....

....

....

....

How do you feel after your practice?

....

....

....

....

....

Date: ....   Duration: ....

How do you feel before your practice?

....

....

....

....

....

How do you feel after your practice?

....

....

....

....

....

Date: ....   Duration: ....

How do you feel before your practice?

....

....

....

....

....

How do you feel after your practice?

....

....

....

....

....

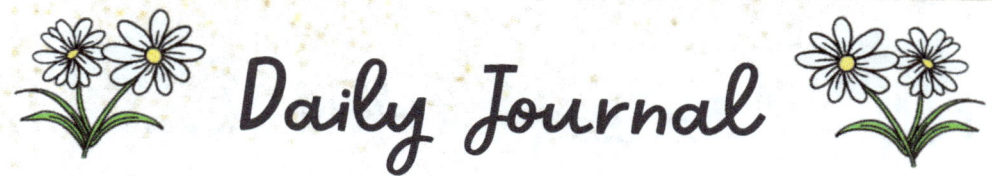

Daily Journal

Daily journaling explores valuable insights into your thoughts, emotions, and experiences, helping you understand and process complex thoughts. This practice fosters self-awareness and identifies patterns for personal growth. In this journal, a few categories are provided to serve as a guide to assist you with your daily journaling.

Top 3 priorities of the day:

....

....

....

Things that motivate you:

....

....

....

Today's goals:

....

....

....

....

....

....

....

Things you choose to focus on today:

....

....

....

....

....

....

3 positive affirmations:

1. ....

....

2. ....

....

3. ....

....

Daily Tasks:

....

....

....

....

....

....

....

....

....

....

How will you rate yourself?

....

....

....

....

Do not forget to:

● ....

● ....

● ....

● ....

● ....

● ....

● ....

● ....

● ....

How do you rate your day? Why?

....

....

....

....

....

....

3 things that you achieved today:

1. ....

2. ....

3. ....

....

Today's highlight:

....

....

....

What were today's challenges?

....

....

....

How did you overcome your challenges today?

....

....

How could you have made today better?

....

....

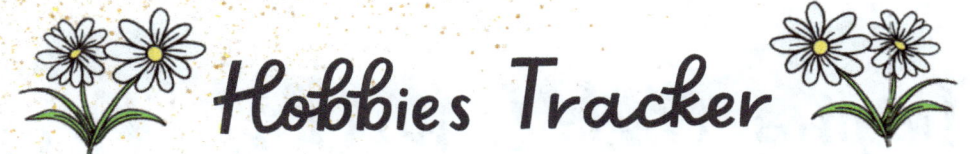

Hobbies Tracker

Engage in activities you enjoy. Whether it's reading, painting, or gardening, hobbies can be therapeutic and provide a break from daily stress.

Date	Hobby	Duration	Notes

Hobbies you are looking forward to trying:

....

....

....

Trying Out Something New

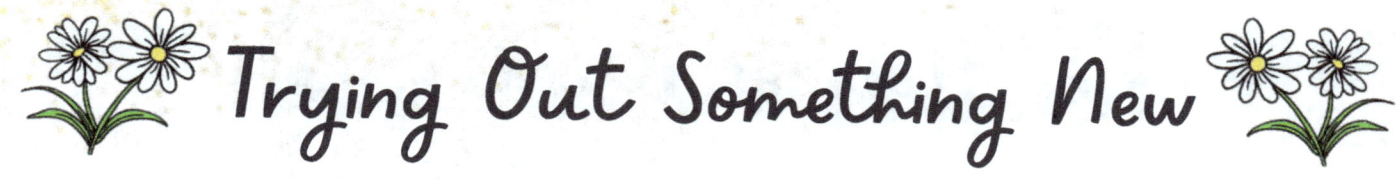

Exploring new activities offers a refreshing break from routine and fosters personal growth. Stepping outside one's comfort zone not only stimulates the mind, but also encourages the development of new skills and perspectives. Choose one of the challenges below that interest you and complete it. After finishing the challenge, jot down your thoughts or experiences. You can repeat this challenge at any time by selecting a different activity or adding new ones.

☐ **Outdoor Activities**

Explore nature through hiking, biking, climbing, running, or other activities.

☐ **Creative Expressions**

Try painting, writing, playing musical instruments, pottery making, and other creative activities to channel emotions and foster self-expression.

☐ **Cooking or Baking**

Try new recipes for a fun and rewarding experience in the kitchen.

☐ **Learning a new skill/ language**

Challenge yourself and boost your confidence.

☐ **Podcasts / Youtube Videos Exploration**

Listen to podcasts or watch Youtube videos on diverse topics to engage your mind and learn something new.

☐ **At Home Spa**

Take a hot bath / scented shower, or applying a facial mask.

☐ **Attend Workshop / Classes**

Attend workshops or classes on topics you're interested in to foster continuous learning and personal growth.

☐ **Travel to New Places**

Explore new destinations to help break away from routine and nurture fresh perspectives.

☐ **Meeting New People**

Participate in gatherings or social events to meet new people or reconnect with old friends to broaden your social circle and boost your mood.

Thought / fears before taking the challenge:

....

....

Thoughts after taking the challenge:

....

....

Other challenges you would love to try:

....

....

Emotional Self-Care

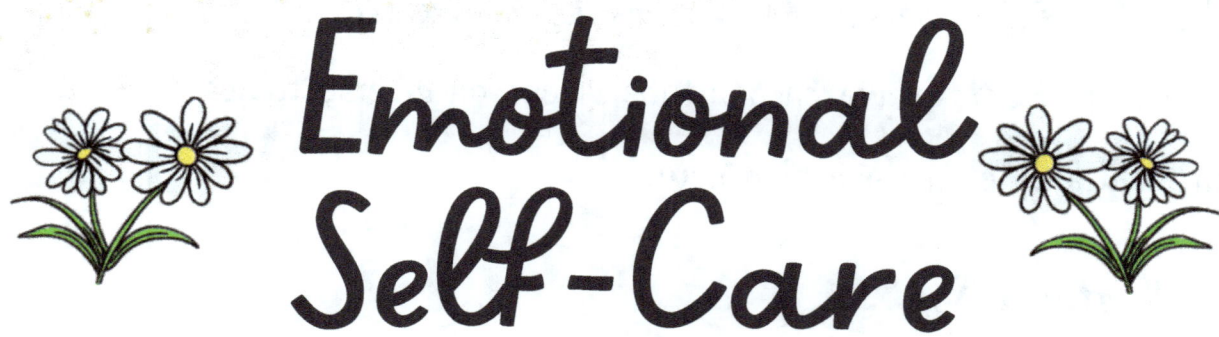

Practicing emotional self-care is the cornerstone to living a fulfilling life, fostering understanding, and managing our emotions effectively. Recognizing and embracing self-compassion cultivates a healthy emotional outlet, helping us build stronger connections with others and achieve lasting emotional harmony.

Notes

....

....

....

....

....

....

....

....

....

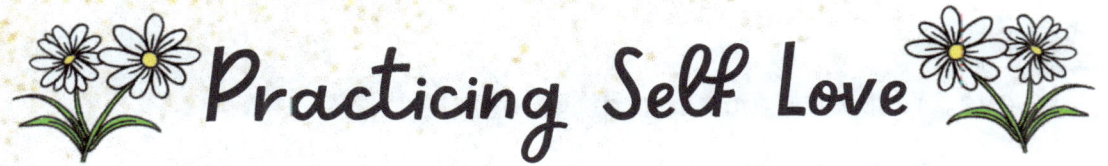 Practicing Self Love

Self-love acts as a powerful shield against criticism and social pressures. A positive self-regard lays a strong foundation for healthier relationships, as individuals who appreciate and value themselves are better equipped to give and receive love. Use the provided checklist daily to assess whether you are giving enough love to yourself. Practice at least five things on the checklist every day, and feel free to add more activities that you can do to show love to yourself.

- ☐ Be kind to yourself. Treat yourself with the same kindness as you would treat a friend.

- ☐ Forgive yourself for your mistakes.

- ☐ Remind yourself of your strengths and capabilities.

- ☐ Learn to say no when necessary. Set clear boundaries in your personal and professional life.

- ☐ Make time for activities that will bring you joy and relaxation.

- ☐ Tell yourself you are amazing.

☐ Love, respect, and accept yourself.

☐ Allow space for your feelings. Give yourself some time to adjust.

☐ Indulge in small pleasure or treat yourself occasionally.

☐ Speak kindly to yourself internally.

☐ Look into the mirror and give yourself a smile.

☐ Learn to say 'I Love You' to yourself.

☐ ....
....

☐ ....
....

☐ ....
....

☐ ....
....

☐ ....
....

☐ ....
....

Letting Go of the Past

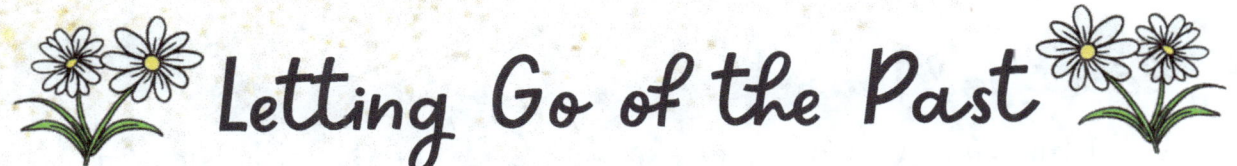

Carrying the weight of past mistakes, regrets, or painful memories can be a constant emotional burden hindering personal growth and happiness. Letting go doesn't diminish one's experience, but promotes healing and reaching a brighter emotional state.

Acceptance

Acknowledge that the past cannot be changed. Understand that dwelling on the past might affect your present and future.

What events or situations from the past are bothering you? (Identifying the root cause can be the first step in addressing and understanding your feelings.)

....

....

....

....

....

What aspects of your past do you have control over, and what aspects do you need to accept? (Recognizing what you can or cannot control can guide you to focus your energy on positive change.)

....

....

....

....

Reflect and Learn

View the past as a learning experience rather than focusing on regrets. Reflecting on the lessons you gained contributes to personal growth.

How have these past experiences affected your current thoughts and behaviors? (Understanding their impact on your current mindset helps identify areas in your life that need healing.)

....

....

....

What lessons have you learned from these experiences? (Seeking wisdom in each encounter turns challenges into opportunities for growth.)

....

....

....

....

How can you reframe your thoughts about the past? (Consider reinterpreting past events in a way that empowers you.)

....

....

....

....

....

....

Forgiveness

View the past as a learning experience rather than focusing on regrets. Reflecting on the lessons you have gained contributes to personal growth.

Are you holding onto any guilt or resentment? (Identifying negative emotions is an essential step in letting go.)

....

....

....

Have you forgiven yourself and others involved?
(Forgiveness is a powerful way to release the grip of the past. Reflect on whether there is a need for forgiveness for yourself and others.)

....

....

....

....

Moving Forward

Set realistic and meaningful goals for the future. Treat yourself with the same kindness as you would treat a friend.

What role does acceptance play in your ability to let go? (Accepting the past with all its imperfections is a powerful catalyst for letting go.)

....

....

....

....

What self-care practices can you apply in your daily life to promote healing? (Engaging in activities that you enjoy can help you relax and contribute to emotional well-being.)

....

....

....

....

What steps can you take to create a more positive future? (Focusing on positive thoughts can prevent you from dwelling on the past.)

....

....

....

....

Reminder

The process of letting go is personal and may take time. Seek help from professionals, family, or friends when struggles persist.

Do you have a support system? (Having a support system is important. Reflect on whether you are reaching out to family, friends, or professionals for assistance when needed.)

....

....

....

....

Turn Negative Thoughts to Positive

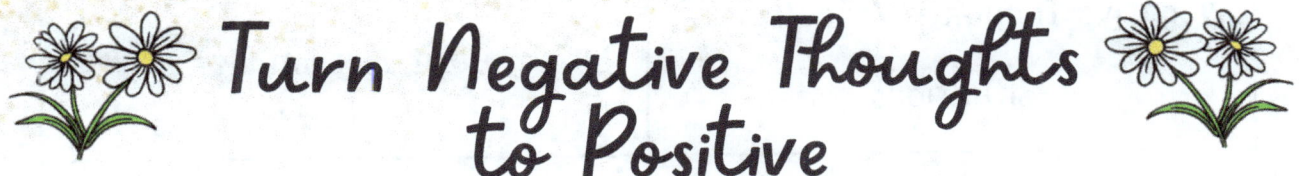

Write down the negative thought, feeling, or situation that is bothering you at the moment. Then, jot down three positive things that can emerge from that negative thought, feeling, or situation. Replacing negative thoughts with positive ones enhances resilience in the face of challenges and boosts happiness, leading to a more fulfilling life.

Negative thoughts / feelings / situations	Positive thoughts
	1. 2. 3.
	1. 2. 3.
	1. 2. 3.

Negative thoughts / feelings / situations	Positive thoughts
	1. 2. 3.
	1. 2. 3.
	1. 2. 3.
	1. 2. 3.
	1. 2. 3.

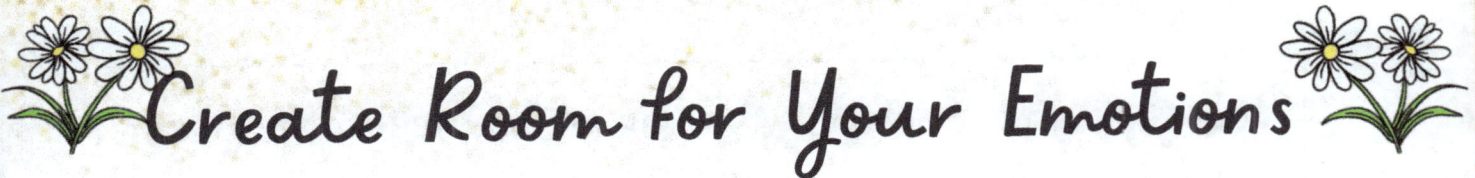

Create Room for Your Emotions

Are you aware of your own emotions? Journal your emotions and write down why you are feeling that way. This practice will help you gain a deeper understanding of yourself and pave the way for personal development.

Your feelings	Rating	Why are you feeling this way?
Happy		
Sad		
Angry		
Excited		
Anxious		
Content		
Stressed		
Calm		

Your feelings	Rating	Why are you feeling this way?
Overwhelmed		
Optimistic		
Pessimistic		
Tired		
Energetic		
Irritated		
Inspired		
Bored		
Surprised		
Relieved		
Confused		
Loved		

Your feelings	Rating	Why are you feeling this way?
Motivated		
Nervous		
Proud		
Disappointed		
Guilty		
Accomplished		
Insecure		
Hopeful		
Apathetic		
Enthusiastic		
Jealous		
Sympathetic		

Your feelings	Rating	Why are you feeling this way?
Regretful		
Frustrated		
Lonely		
Disgusted		

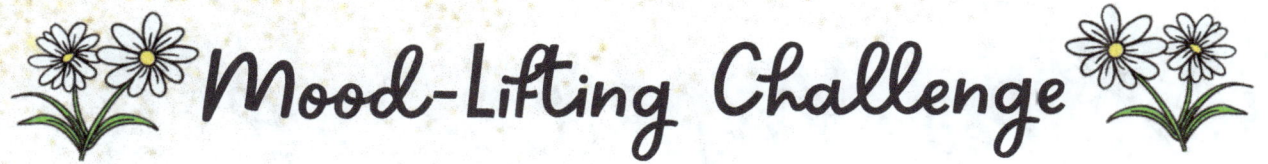

Mood-Lifting Challenge

Try one or more activities in this mood-lifting challenge when you are having a bad day or feeling low. Take note of the activities that uplift your mood and make you feel better. Practice that activity or thought process to instantly uplift your mood the next time you are experiencing negative feelings.

Walk in nature	Cook your favorite meal	Practice positive affirmations
Perform breathing exercises	Look back at old videos / photos	Listen to your favorite music
Journal your thoughts	Create a vision board	Write about 10 things that you love

Hobbies you are looking forward to try:

....

....

....

....

....

....

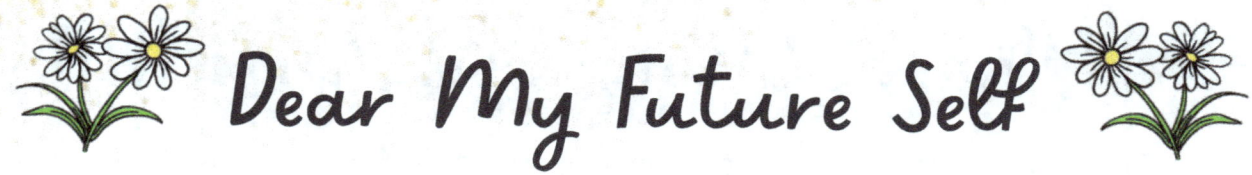

Dear My Future Self

Take a moment to pen a letter to your future self. In doing so, you gift yourself the therapeutic balm of self-reflection, set the compass for your aspirations, and create a timeless connection with the resilient, evolving person you are becoming. Happy writing, and may your future self thank you for this act of kindness and self-care.

Dear future self,

....

....

....

....

....

....

....

....

....

....

....

....

....

....

Social Self-Care

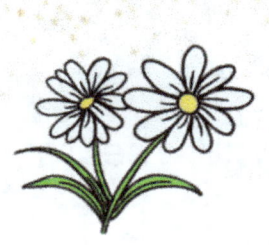 

Social interaction is essential as a source of emotional and mental well-being. By spending time with supportive friends and family, we can openly express our thoughts and feelings, reduce stress, and enhance our sense of belonging. Besides boosting our self-esteem, building connections and nurturing relationships also provide valuable support during challenging times.

Notes

....

....

....

....

....

....

....

....

....

Setting Boundaries

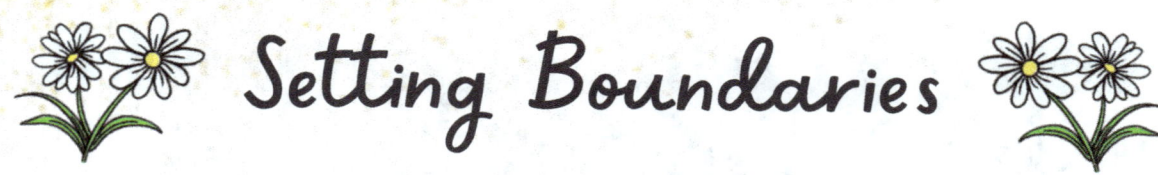

Setting boundaries is a great way to protect your mental and emotional well-being. Besides that, setting clear boundaries also contributes to healthier and more fulfilling relationships.

Type of boundary	What are the boundaries you want to make?	How can you establish the boundaries?	Note to self
Time			
Personal space			
Social events			

Type of boundary	What are the boundaries you would like to make?	How can you establish the boundaries?	Note to self
Communication style			
Emotional support			
Privacy			
Social media			
Work-life balance			

Letting Go of People

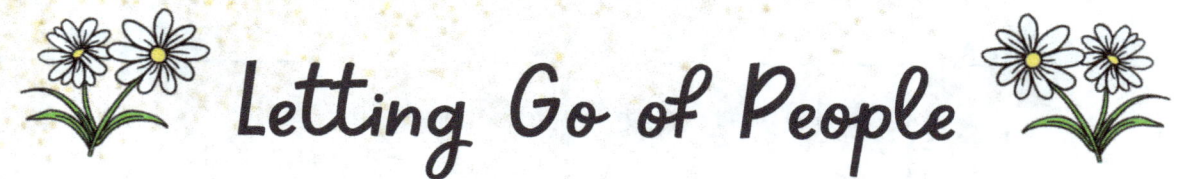

In relationships that no longer serve your best interest or even harms you physically or mentally, letting go becomes a courageous act of self-preservation. It allows space for healing, self-discovery, and the pursuit of healthier relationships. Take time to answer the questions provided, allowing yourself to reflect and analyze whether now is the right time to let someone go.

Are you currently in any relationships that are hurting you?

....

....

....

....

If so, what is the impact of these relationships on your well-being?

....

....

....

....

Did you set clear boundaries with people who negatively affected your mental and emotional health?

....

....

....

....

Did you communicate your boundaries assertively and diplomatically while expressing your needs and expectations to the person?

....
....
....
....

Does the person understand and respect your boundaries?

....
....
....
....
....

What did you do or tell that person if they crossed your boundaries?

....
....
....
....
....

Will you forgive them if this is the first time they crossed your boundaries? If so, how often can you tolerate it before you find it intolerable?

....
....
....
....
....

What are some behaviors that would cause you to let go of the other person if they exhibit them?

....

....

....

....

....

What would the process of letting that person go look like?

....

....

....

....

....

How will you be kind to yourself in this situation?

....

....

....

....

How would you give yourself and the other person time and space to reflect, adjust, and adapt to the changes in the process of letting go?

....

....

....

....

....

How would you seek support from family, friends, or professional therapists if you encounter any challenges in this process of letting go?

....
....
....
....
....
....
....

How would you periodically assess how the changes are impacting your life and well-being?

....
....
....
....
....
....
....
....

How would you celebrate the positive changes you have made?

....
....
....
....
....
....
....

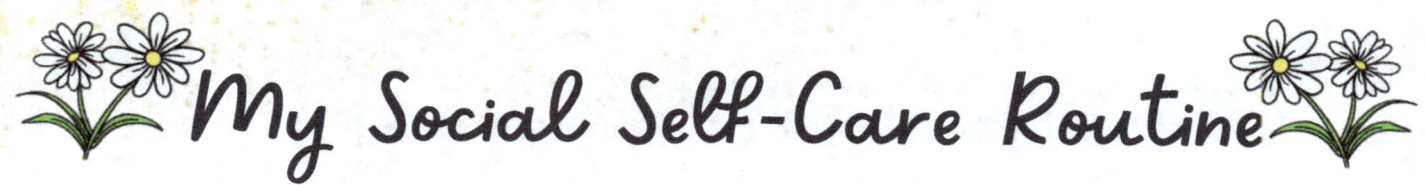

My Social Self-Care Routine

The things listed in this checklist act as a guide to help you maintain a healthy and happy social self-care. Check whether you did at least five things from the list to make sure you are on the right path. Feel free to add in the things that are essential to your routine.

- ☐ Call / talk with family and friends.

- ☐ Invest time in cultivating new relationships.

- ☐ Improve your communication skill.

- ☐ Practice active listening to understand others better.

- ☐ Learn to say no when necessary.

- ☐ Establish healthy boundaries to protect your emotional well-being.

- ☐ Spend quality time with loved ones.

- ☐ Engage in activities with others that bring joy and strengthen relationships.

☐ Meet like-minded individuals to expand your social circle.

☐ Don't be afraid to express your authentic self.

☐ Share your thoughts and feelings with trusted friends.

☐ Take breaks from digital devices to focus on face-to-face interactions.

☐ Put yourself in others' shoes to understand their perspectives.

☐ Show empathy and compassion in your interactions.

☐ Acknowledge and celebrate your accomplishments with friends and family.

☐ Reflect on your social interactions and relationships regularly. Identify areas for improvement and personal growth.

☐ Address conflict openly and constructively. Seek resolutions that strengthen relationships rather than create distance.

☐ Embrace solitude and use it as an opportunity for self-reflection and personal growth.

- ☐ Adjust your social activities based on your needs and feelings.

- ☐ Check in with yourself regularly and assess your social well-being.

- ☐ Participate in clubs, organizations, or social group events that align with your interests.

- ☐ Avoid toxic relationships that drain your energy.

- ☐ Be present during social interactions.

- ☐ ....

- ☐ ....

- ☐ ....

- ☐ ....

- ☐ ....

- ☐ ....

- ☐ ....

- ☐ ....

- ☐ ....

Alone Time Planner

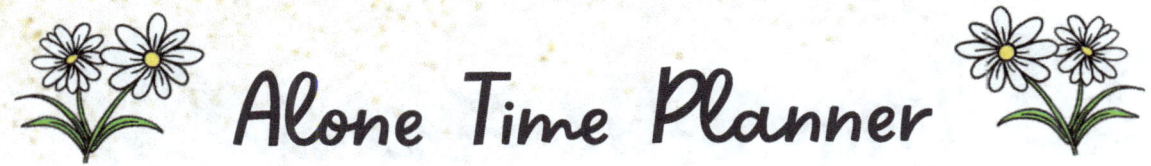

Below is a simple table for you to plan some alone time for yourself. Make sure to use the table or modify it to suit your needs to plan some quality alone time that is enjoyable for you.

Date	Time	Activity	Notes

My Social Planner

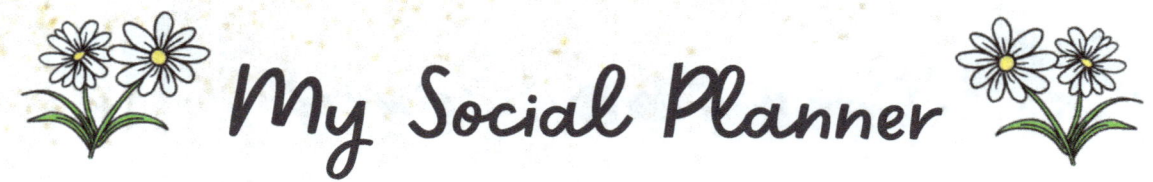

Planning and organizing your social interactions can help you prioritize your social goals. The table provided is an example you can use. Feel free to customize it according to your preferences.

Date			
Day			
Time			
Activity / event			
Venue / location			
Purpose / goal			
People involved			
Notes / reflections			

Date			
Day			
Time			
Activity / event			
Venue / location			
Purpose / goal			
People involved			
Notes / reflections			

Spiritual Self-Care

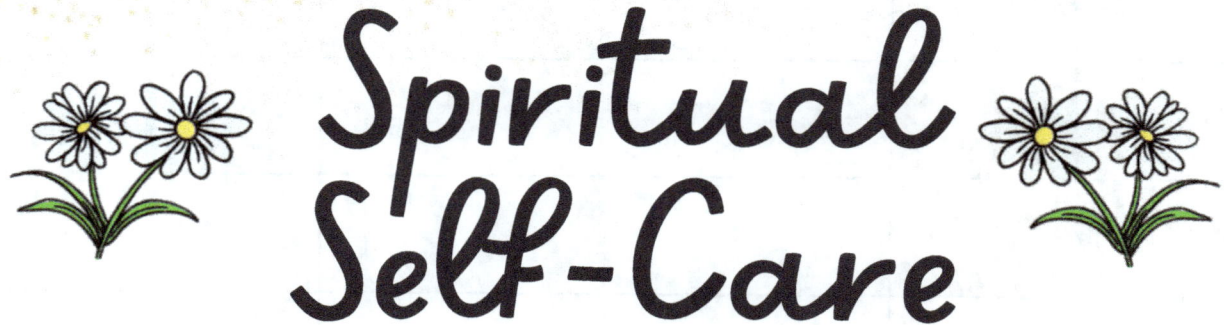

Spiritual self-care is a practice that nurtures our inner essence by delving into personal beliefs, values, and life's purpose. Tending to our spiritual needs allows us to connect with our inner selves, find meaning, foster fulfillment, and cultivate a sense of harmony.

Notes

....

....

....

....

....

....

....

....

Spiritual Self-Care Routine

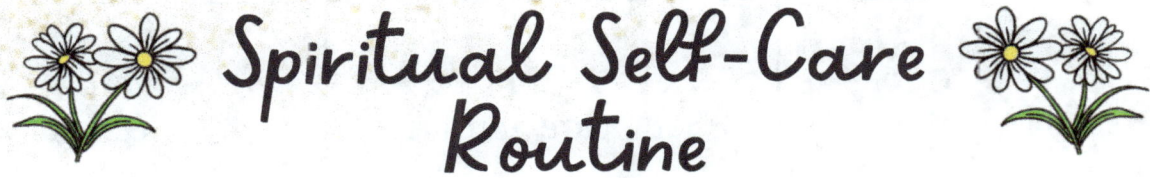

This journal provides a table for you to write down your current goals for spiritual self-care. This table can also help you plan and manage your spiritual self-care routines. Feel free to customize the table based on what resonates with you.

What does your spiritual self-care look like right now?

....
....
....
....
....
....

Are you satisfied with your current spiritual self-care? Why?

....
....
....
....
....
....

Time slot	Self-care routine	Goals
Morning		
Midday		
Afternoon		
Evening		
Night		
Before bed		

Sacred Gatherings

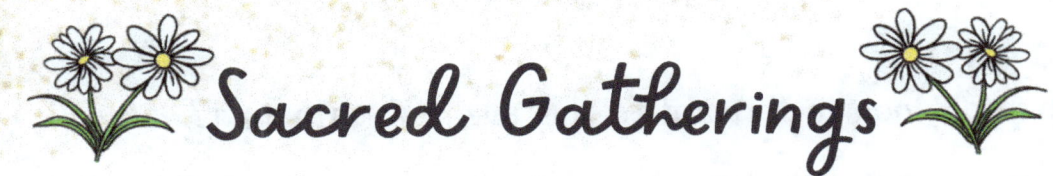

Participating in meaningful events that resonate with you can help you connect with like-minded people. Furthermore, engaging in such events fosters a sense of community and support. Here's a detailed journal that you can use to record your thoughts and feelings toward your fulfillment and purpose.

Type of event / gathering: ....

What is the purpose of this event / gathering?

....

....

....

What is the date and time for this event?

....

....

....

Does this event / gathering have a theme? If yes, what is the theme?

....

....

....

Are you looking forward to this event / gathering? Why?

....

....

....

....

What are your thoughts on this event / gathering after attending it? Why?

....

....

....

....

What lessons did you learn from participating in this event / gathering?

....

....

....

What can you do to perform better at this event / gathering?

....

....

....

If this event / gathering is going to be held again in the future, would you be interested in participating again? Why?

....

....

....

Gratitude Journal

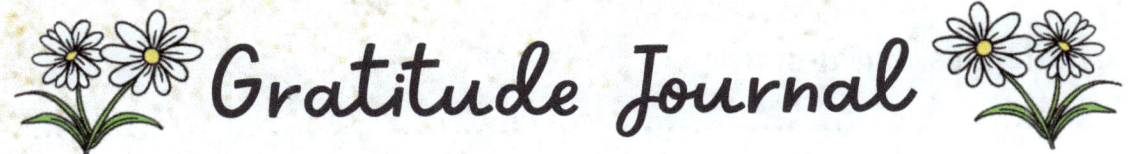

Gratitude is essential, as it acts as a channel for connecting with a deeper sense of purpose and meaning. Cultivating gratitude involves acknowledging both the significant and minor blessings that contribute to one's life. Take a moment to write down at least three things that you are grateful for in each of the mentioned areas.

Date: ....

I am truly grateful for ....

   1. Morning reflections:

....

....

....

....

   2. Health and well-being:

....

....

....

....

   3. Relationships:

....

....

....

....

4. Challenges and growth:

....
....
....

5. Nature and surroundings:

....
....
....

6. Accomplishments and achievements:

....
....
....

7. Random acts of kindness:

....
....
....

8. Moments of joy:

....
....
....

9. Reflections of the day:

....
....
....

10. Evening appreciation:

....
....
....

Visualization

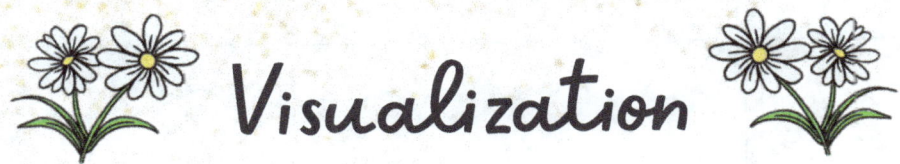

Through the practice of visualization, individuals can create mental images that represent their goals, aspirations, and desired states of being. This process reinforces spiritual intentions, acts as a catalyst for manifesting positive energy, and attracts spiritual abundance. Fill in the table provided to track your visualization practices and identify areas for improvement in the next sessions.

Date			
Duration			
Visualization topics			
Thoughts before visualization			
Thoughts after visualization			
What you can improve			
Notes			

Date			
Duration			
Visualization topics			
Thoughts before visualization			
Thoughts after visualization			
What you can improve			
Notes			

Spiritual Self-Care Checklist

Check off as many practices as possible each day to ensure you are on the right path in practicing and maintaining a healthy spiritual routine. Feel free to add to the checklist.

- ☐ Begin the day with gratitude. Acknowledge the blessings in your life.

- ☐ Engage in brief meditation / visualization to center your mind and cultivate inner peace.

- ☐ Spend time in prayer. Connect with your spiritual beliefs and seek guidance.

- ☐ Practice positive affirmations to foster a mindset of self-love and empowerment.

- ☐ Practice deep breathing exercises to promote relaxation and mindfulness.

- ☐ Read inspirational and motivational texts or literature.

- ☐ Perform acts of kindness to foster a sense of compassion and connection.

- ☐ Journal your thoughts and emotions to promote self-awareness and reflection.

- ☐ Attend spiritual gatherings or community events to share and strengthen your beliefs.

- ☐ Embrace moments of silence to listen to your inner self and connect with your intuition.

- ☐ Practice faith.

- ☐ Feel the present moment.

- ☐ Spend some time with nature.

- ☐ ....

- ☐ ....

- ☐ ....

- ☐ ....

- ☐ ....

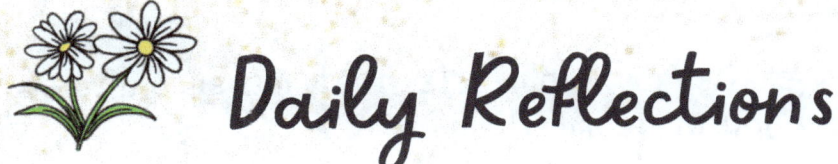 

Daily Reflections

Regularly reviewing your day can provide valuable insights into your daily life, helping you make positive changes and improvements over time.

Date: ....

How did you feel when you first woke up?

....
....
....

How did your current morning routine set the tone for your day?

....
....
....

What tasks or goals did you complete successfully?

....
....
....

Were there any challenges / obstacles that you encountered today? How did you overcome them?

···
···
···

Did you engage in your self-care activities today? If not, why?

···
···
···

How did your self-care activities contribute to your well-being?

···
···
···

How do you rate your day today?

···
···
···

What can you do to make tomorrow better?

···
···
···

Physical Self-Care

Exercise, balanced nutrition, and proper rest shape our physical health. Regular exercise keeps our muscles in peak condition, while a healthy, balanced diet provides nutrients for our bodies to function optimally. Adequate rest allows our bodies to rejuvenate and recover. Caring for these three areas promotes a healthier, happier self.

Notes

....

....

....

....

....

....

....

....

Your Goal for Physical Health

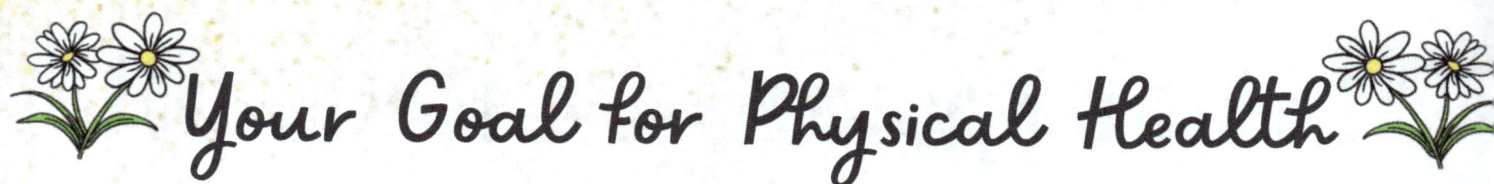

Taking great care of our bodies will contribute to physical fitness and has positive effects on mental and emotional health. Write down your goals for all the mentioned areas to serve as motivation for consistently practicing good physical self-care.

Regular exercise

Did you incorporate exercise routines to include stretching, strength training, and cardio?

....
....
....
....

Did you engage in at least 75 minutes of exercise per week?

....
....
....
....

Do you include activities that you enjoy to make exercise a sustainable part of your routine?

....
....
....

Balanced Nutrition

Did you consume a well-rounded diet rich in fruits, vegetables, grains, lean proteins, and healthy fats?

....

....

....

Did you stay hydrated by drinking an adequate amount of water throughout the day?

....

....

....

Are you mindful of portion sizes to maintain a healthy weight?

....

....

....

Adequate Sleep

Do you sleep 7-9 hours of quality sleep each night?

....

....

....

Do you establish a consistent sleep schedule and create a relaxing bedtime routine?

....

....

....

Hygiene Practices

Do you maintain good personal hygiene?

....

....

....

What is your routine?

....

....

....

Stress Management

Do you practice stress-reducing activities such as yoga, deep breathing, or meditation?

....

....

....

Do you allocate time for hobbies and activities that will bring you joy?

....

....

....

....

Regular Health Check-Ups

Do you schedule routine medical check-ups and screenings to detect potential health issues early?

....
....
....

Do your vaccinations and preventive care stay up-to-date?

....
....
....

Posture Awareness

Are you mindful of your posture, especially if you have a sedentary lifestyle?

....
....
....

Do you take breaks to stretch and move around throughout the day?

....
....
....

Avoid Harmful Substances

Do you minimize the consumption of alcohol, tobacco, and other harmful substances?

....

....

....

Relaxation Techniques

Do you incorporate relaxation techniques such as taking hot baths, massages, or aromatherapy to unwind?

....

....

....

Proper Clothing and Footwear

Do you wear appropriate clothing and footwear during exercise to prevent injuries and discomfort?

....

....

....

Listen to Your Body

Do you pay attention to your body's signals?

....

....

....

If you feel pain or fatigue, do you rest and seek professional

advice if needed?

....

....

....

Meal Planner

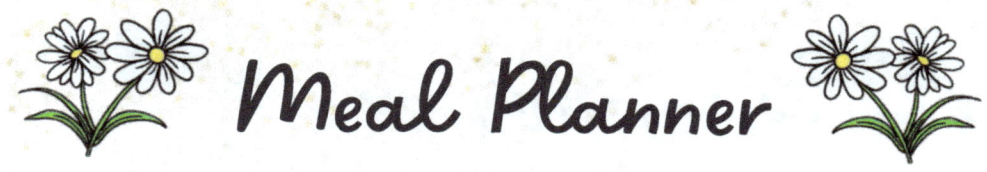

Prioritizing a healthy meal is important to provide the bodies with essential nutrients and energy. A well-balanced and nutritious diet keeps our bodies functioning optimally, strengthens our immune system, and sustains energy level. Making mindful choices about what we eat is a proactive way to nurture our bodies and maintain our health. Feel free to customize the table according to your requirements.

Day	Mon	Tue	Wed	Thu	Fri	Sat	Sun
Breakfast							
Lunch							
Dinner							
Snacks							
Notes							
Shopping list							

Day	Mon	Tue	Wed	Thu	Fri	Sat	Sun
Breakfast							
Lunch							
Dinner							
Snacks							
Notes							
Shopping list							

Health Tracker

Date:

What time did you go to bed last night?

....

What time did you wake up this morning?

....

How many hours did you sleep last night?

....

What is your heart rate?

Morning: ....   Afternoon:

....

Evening: ....   Night:

....

How many steps have you taken today?

....

What is your weight today?

....

What is your calorie intake today?

....

What type of exercise did you do today?

....

How long did you exercise today?

....

What is your energy level today?

....

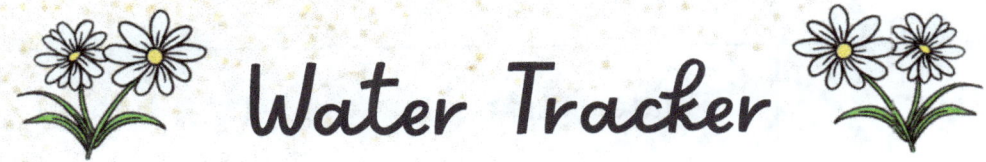

Water Tracker

Adequate hydration is essential for numerous bodily functions. Water plays a vital role in regulating body temperature, aiding digestion, and transporting nutrients throughout the system. Sufficient water intake is a powerful practice to ensure our bodies operate at their best and foster overall physical vitality. The common guideline suggests drinking eight 8-ounce glasses of water daily. Track your water intake to ensure you stay hydrated consistently.

Day	Water intake	Notes
Monday		
Tuesday		
Wednesday		
Thursday		
Friday		
Saturday		
Sunday		

Day	Water intake	Notes
Monday		
Tuesday		
Wednesday		
Thursday		
Friday		
Saturday		
Sunday		

Day	Water intake	Notes
Monday		
Tuesday		
Wednesday		
Thursday		
Friday		
Saturday		
Sunday		

A Grateful Farewell and Wishes for Well-Being

As you conclude this self-care journal, I want to extend my heartfelt gratitude to each reader who embarked on this journey of self-discovery and consciousness with me. May the practices and insights gained from this journal become an enduring companion on your path to a healthier and more balanced life. I wish you all the best as you continue to nurture yourself, live intentionally, and cultivate a flourishing life filled with joy and fulfillment. Take good care of yourselves, and may your day be blessed with abundance and well-deserved self-care.

Remember, self-care is an ongoing journey - it's a marathon not a sprint.